THE ELDERLY DIET COOKBOOK:

Nourishing Golden years

Paul McKinney

© 2023 Paul McKinney

All rights reserved. No part of this book may be reproduced or transmitted in any form or by any means, electronic or mechanical, including photocopying, recording, or any other information storage and retrieval system, without written permission from the author, except for the inclusion of brief quotations in a review.

TABLE OF CONTENTS

I. Introduction to the Elderly Diet Cookbook
- The significance of nutrition to the Elderly population
- Common health problems that older people face and how diet can help
- Overview of the foods in the cookbook

II. Recipes for Breakfast, lunch and dinner

- Why the elderly need to eat breakfast
- Recipes for quick and filling breakfasts, with options for those who have dietary restrictions or difficulty chewing
- Tips for making breakfast preparation and consumption easier for the elderly
- Recipes for quick and healthy lunch and dinner options, including options for seniors with dietary restrictions or chewing issues
- Tips for making it easier for seniors to prepare and consume meals
- Discussion of portion sizes and meal planning for the elderly that is balanced

III. Desserts and Snacks

- why snacks and desserts can be important for the elderly

- Recipes for easy, healthy snacks and desserts, including options for those with dietary restrictions or difficulty chewing
- Tips for making the preparation and consumption of snacks and desserts easier for the elderly

IV. Healthy Eating and Meal Planning for Older People
- Elderly meal planning and healthy eating habits
- Tips for elderly grocery shopping and food storage
- Ideas for getting family members and caregivers involved in meal planning and preparations

Introduction to the Elderly Diet Cookbook

Our nutritional requirements shift with age. The elderly have special dietary needs, so it's important to make sure they get the right nutrients to keep their health and well-being. The Elderly Diet Cookbook was created with seniors in mind, making it easy to prepare nutritious meals for them.

Nutrition is important for seniors because it can help prevent and treat diseases like diabetes, heart disease, and osteoporosis. A healthy diet can also help you feel better, have more energy, and think better.

A variety of recipes suitable for seniors and simple to prepare are included in this cookbook. It has options for people who have trouble chewing and following dietary restrictions like low-sodium or low-fat diets.

Seniors can get the vitamins and minerals they need to stay healthy from the recipes, which are balanced and packed with nutrients.

In the accompanying sections, we will give recipes to breakfast, lunch, and supper, as well as tidbits and sweets.

We will likewise examine good dieting propensities and dinner arranging procedures for the older to assist them with keeping up with their wellbeing and freedom.

The significance of nutrition to the Elderly population

The significance of nourishment for the old populace couldn't possibly be more significant. Our bodies change as we get older, which can affect how much food we need. For instance, our digestion dials back, and our bodies become less productive at engrossing supplements. What's more, more seasoned grown-ups may have a decreased craving, which can prompt unhealthiness.

The elderly population needs to eat well to keep their health and well-being. Diabetes, heart disease, and osteoporosis are just a few of the chronic diseases it can help to prevent and treat. In addition, adequate nutrition can support cognitive function, enhance mood, and increase energy levels.

A healthy diet can support healthy weight maintenance in addition to providing the necessary nutrients. This is important because obesity can raise the risk of many diseases, such as diabetes and heart disease. On the other hand, being underweight can make falls and fractures more likely.

Overall, the elderly need to eat a well-balanced, nutrient-dense diet to keep their health and independence. The Elderly Diet Cookbook was created so that seniors can get the nutrition they need with easy, nutritious meals.

Common health problems that older people face and how diet can help

The elderly population is more likely than younger adults to have health problems. Seniors frequently face the following health problems:

- Malnutrition: Malnutrition is a prevalent problem among the elderly, as previously mentioned. A number of health issues, including fatigue, weakness, and a weakened immune system, may result from this.

- Chronic conditions: Chronic diseases like diabetes, heart disease, and osteoporosis are more common in older adults. These conditions can be managed and complications avoided with a healthy diet.

- Cognitive impairment: A healthy diet can support cognitive function, prevent or slow down dementia, and cognitive decline is a natural part of aging.

- Problems with the digestive system: Constipation and acid reflux are two common digestive issues that plague many senior citizens. These problems can be prevented and managed with the help of a healthy diet high in fiber.

- Interactions between drugs: Multiple medications are often taken by older people, which can make it harder for nutrients to be absorbed. A solid eating routine can assist with guaranteeing that seniors are getting the supplements they need to help their wellbeing.

The elderly population's overall health and well-being can be improved and these health issues managed by diet. Recipes from The Elderly Diet Cookbook address these issues and provide seniors with the nutrients they need to stay healthy. Seniors can manage chronic health conditions, maintain cognitive function, and enhance their overall quality of life by eating a well-balanced, nutrient-dense diet.

Overview of the foods in the cookbook

The Elderly Diet Cookbook contains a variety of nutrient-dense, simple-to-prepare, and senior-friendly foods. The recipes have been created with seniors in mind so that they can get the right amount of the nutrients they need to stay healthy. The cookbook contains a variety of foods, including the following:

- Products of the soil: Vitamins, minerals, and fiber can all be found in these important sources. Smoothies, soups, salads, and stir-fries with a variety of fruits and vegetables are all included in the cookbook.

- Grains whole: These can help maintain healthy blood sugar levels and are a good source of fiber. The cookbook incorporates recipes for cereal, entire grain bread, and quinoa bowls.

- Lean proteins: Protein is necessary for supporting immune function and maintaining muscle mass. The cookbook incorporates recipes for chicken, fish, beans, and tofu.

- Alternatives to dairy: Many seniors have trouble digesting dairy products or are lactose intolerant. Almond milk and tofu are two examples of calcium-rich alternatives in the cookbook.

- wholesome fats: A healthy diet should include fats, but it's important to choose the right kinds. There are recipes in the book for healthy fats like olive oil, nuts, and seeds.

- Low-sodium and low-fat choices: A low-fat or low-sodium diet is one restriction that many seniors adhere to. Recipes for these dietary requirements are included in the cookbook.

In general, the Elderly Diet Cookbook includes a variety of scrumptious and healthy recipes made just for seniors. Seniors can maintain their health and wellness while also enjoying delicious meals by incorporating a variety of whole foods, lean proteins, and healthy fats.

Recipes for Breakfast, lunch and dinner

Most people agree that breakfast is the most important meal of the day, especially the elderly. Seniors can get the energy and nutrients they need to start their day off right by eating a healthy breakfast. There are a number of breakfast recipes in The Elderly Diet Cookbook that are both nutrient-dense and simple to prepare. Some examples include:

- Oats for the night: This is a breakfast option that can be made the night before and is easy and delicious. In a mason jar, combine rolled oats, almond milk, chia seeds, and your preferred toppings, such as fruits and nuts, and refrigerate for the night. You'll be prepared for the day with a nutritious and filling breakfast in the morning.

- Omelet of vegetables: A great way to consume vegetables early in the day is this. Sautee spinach, mushrooms, and onions in a non-stick skillet and pour in beaten eggs. Sprinkle some grated cheese on top and cook until the eggs are set. For a healthy and filling breakfast, pair it with toast made with whole grains.

- Plaquet of yogurt: When combined with granola and berries, Greek yogurt is a delicious and nutrient-dense breakfast option. It is also an excellent source of protein and calcium. In a glass or bowl, layer your favorite granola, Greek yogurt, and mixed berries.

- Bowl of smoothies: Smoothie bowls are a great way to get your morning nutrients and fiber. A scoop of protein powder, frozen berries, spinach, almond milk, and the mixture should be smooth. Layer sliced fruit, nuts, and seeds on top of the smoothie in a serving bowl.

- Pancakes with whole grains: Hotcakes can in any case be a solid breakfast choice when made with entire grain flour and presented with new foods grown from the ground dab of Greek yogurt. Cook on a nonstick griddle with whole wheat flour, baking powder, milk, and an egg. Serve with Greek yogurt and fresh berries.

The Elderly Diet Cookbook contains a wide range of delicious and nutritious options, including these breakfast recipes. Seniors can maintain their energy levels and prepare for a productive and enjoyable day by starting the day with a healthy and balanced breakfast.

Why the elderly need to eat breakfast

Breakfast is an essential meal for all people, but the elderly need it the most. Our bodies lose their ability to absorb nutrients from food as we get older, which can lead to a decrease in appetite.

As a result, seniors may not receive all of the nutrients they require from their meals, and skipping breakfast can exacerbate this problem.

For seniors, skipping breakfast can have a number of negative effects on their health. For instance, it may result in a drop in blood sugar levels, which can cause confusion, fatigue, and dizziness.

Malnutrition, which can have serious effects on one's overall health and well-being, may also be more likely to occur as a result.

Seniors can get the nutrients and energy they need to start their day right by eating a healthy breakfast.

Additionally, it may assist in regulating appetite and preventing later overeating.

Compared to seniors who skip breakfast, those who eat a healthy breakfast have better cognitive function, mood stability, and overall health, according to studies.

In conclusion, seniors should eat breakfast because it can give them the nutrients and energy they need to start the day off right, prevent bad health outcomes, and improve their overall health and well-being.

Recipes for quick and filling breakfasts, with options for those who have dietary restrictions or difficulty chewing

Here are some quick and filling breakfast ideas for seniors that take into account dietary restrictions and difficulty chewing:

- Eggs lightly scrambled: Although scrambled eggs are a great source of protein, chewing them can be difficult for seniors. Soft scrambled eggs are an alternative that are easier to swallow and chew because they are softer. Over low heat, cook the eggs until they are light and fluffy, stirring frequently.

- Greek yogurt with nuts, mashed banana: Greek yogurt is an incredible wellspring of protein and calcium, and pounded banana adds normal pleasantness and fiber. For extra crunch and healthy fats, garnish with chopped nuts.

- Soft fruit overnight oats: For seniors who have trouble chewing, overnight oats are a great choice. Allow the rolled oats, milk (or an alternative), and chia seeds to sit overnight in a bowl or jar. For added nutrition in the morning, top with soft fruits like chopped peaches or berries.

- Pudding with chia seeds: Chia seeds are high in fiber, protein, and solid fats, and they can be ready as a pudding that is not difficult to eat. Chia seeds should be mixed with milk or another liquid, and they should be refrigerated overnight. Top with chopped fruit, nuts, or granola in the morning.

- Banana pancakes without gluten: Flapjacks can be made sans gluten by utilizing a blend of sans gluten flours like almond flour and coconut flour. Squash a ready banana and blend it in with the flapjack hitter for added regular pleasantness. For a balanced meal, serve with fresh fruit and Greek yogurt.

- Scrambled vegetables and tofu: A tofu and vegetable scramble is a healthy and simple option for seniors who eat vegetarian or vegan. In a non-stick pan, sauté onions, peppers, and mushrooms before adding tofu and cooking until heated through. Add flavor by seasoning with herbs and spices.

- These breakfast ideas are simple to make, nutritious, and take into account senior citizens' dietary restrictions and chewing difficulties. Seniors can maintain their energy levels and prepare themselves for a productive and enjoyable day by starting the day with a nutritious breakfast.

Tips for making breakfast preparation and consumption easier for the elderly

Some elderly people find it difficult to prepare and consume breakfast. For your convenience, here are some suggestions:

- Make breakfast easy: Choose easy breakfast options that don't take a lot of time to prepare or clean up. Seniors will find the procedure less stressful as a result.

- Pre-segment food: To make it easier for seniors to prepare and serve breakfast, think about portioning meals and ingredients in advance. For ease of cooking, for instance, chop vegetables ahead of time for an omelet or portion oatmeal into microwave-safe containers.

- Utilize simple to-utilize apparatuses: Choose kitchen appliances that don't require a lot of manual dexterity and are simple to operate. A single-serve coffee maker, microwave, or toaster, for instance, may be easier to use for seniors than a stove or traditional coffee pot.

- Provide tools that adapt: Think about giving seniors adaptive utensils, like spoons with thicker handles or angled utensils that make it easier to reach food.

- Check the lighting: To lessen the likelihood of slips and falls and other accidents, ensure that the eating area and kitchen are well-lit.

- Choose foods high in nutrients: To help seniors maintain their energy levels throughout the day, choose foods that are rich in nutrients and a good source of protein, vitamins, and minerals.

- Make eating a social encounter: Seniors should be encouraged to eat breakfast with friends or family. This can assist in making the process more pleasurable and provide social interaction, both of which are crucial for one's overall well-being.

You can help make breakfast preparation and consumption easier and more enjoyable for the elderly population by following these tips.

Recipes for quick and healthy lunch and dinner options, including options for seniors with dietary restrictions or chewing issues

- Vegetables and chicken slow-cooked: A quick and easy way to prepare a nutritious and flavorful meal is to slow cook chicken and vegetables. In a slow cooker, simply add the chicken, vegetables like potatoes and carrots, broth, and cook on low for 6 to 8 hours.

- A salad of tuna and avocado: Avocado adds healthy fats and nutrients to tuna salad, which is a great source of protein. For extra creaminess, combine mashed avocado, chopped celery, and Greek yogurt with canned tuna.

- Squash soup: Seniors who have difficulty chewing should try lentil soup. The soup can be seasoned with herbs and spices to add flavor, and lentils are a good source of protein and fiber. Whole-grain bread on the side provides additional nutrition.

- Salmon and vegetables grilled: Omega-3 fatty acids, which are important for heart health, are abundant in grilled salmon. For more nutrients, serve with grilled vegetables like bell peppers and zucchini.

- Chili with sweet potatoes and black beans: Black beans and sweet potatoes are both good sources of protein and fiber, and they can be combined to make a tasty and healthy chili. For more flavor, add chili powder, diced onions, and tomatoes.

- Tofu-based vegetarian stir-fry: Stir-fry is a quick and simple dish that can be altered to include a variety of vegetables and protein sources. For a veggie lover choice, pan sear tofu with vegetables like broccoli, mushrooms, and carrots, and serve over earthy colored rice for added fiber.

These suggestions for lunch and dinner are nutritious, simple to prepare, and take into account senior citizens' dietary restrictions and chewing difficulties. By giving seniors supplement thick dinners that are not difficult to eat, you can assist with supporting their general wellbeing and prosperity.

Tips for making it easier for seniors to prepare and consume meals

The following are some suggestions for making it easier for seniors to prepare and consume meals:

- Make meals in advance: Preparing meals and shopping for groceries can be made simpler with meal planning. Make a weekly meal plan with a variety of nutrient-dense foods in mind.

- Make use of pre-made ingredients: During meal preparation, pre-prepared ingredients can save time and energy. Reduce preparation time by utilizing pre-chopped vegetables or cooked meats.

- Decide simple to-utilize apparatuses: Seniors may find it easier to prepare meals with kitchen appliances that are simple to operate. Instead of a stove or oven, think about using an electric kettle, microwave, or slow cooker.

- Utilize adaptable tools: Seniors may find it easier to eat with the help of adaptive utensils. Use utensils with thicker handles or angled utensils to reach food more easily.

- Check the lighting: Legitimate lighting can diminish the gamble of mishaps and falls during dinner readiness and utilization. Make sure the dining area and kitchen have adequate lighting.

- Encourage eating with others: When you eat with others, you can enjoy mealtimes more and get social interaction, which is important for your overall health. Seniors should be encouraged to eat with friends or family.

- Make food more appealing: A senior's appetite can be affected by how meals are presented. To enhance the visual appeal of your meals, think about using garnishes and plates in vibrant colors.

- Make meals smaller and more frequent: Large meals may be difficult for seniors to consume. To ensure adequate nutrition, think about serving smaller, more frequent meals throughout the day.

You can make meal preparation and consumption for seniors easier by following these tips. Giving supplement thick feasts that are not difficult to eat can assist with supporting their general wellbeing and prosperity.

Discussion of portion sizes and meal planning for the elderly that is balanced

When it comes to meal planning for the elderly, it is essential to take into account portion sizes and balance.

The following are some pointers for elderly meal planning and portion control:

- Choose foods high in nutrients: Foods that are high in nutrients offer a lot of nutrition for a small amount of calories. Whole grains, lean proteins, vegetables, fruits, and low-fat dairy products are examples of these. By choosing these foods, seniors avoid overeating and get the nutrients they need.

- Make use of small plates: Utilizing more modest plates can assist with controlling part estimates. A smaller plate can give the impression that there is more food on it, which can make seniors feel better about eating smaller portions.

- Macronutrients in balance: Carbohydrates, proteins, and fats are examples of macronutrients—nutrients that the body requires in greater quantities. A variety of these nutrients should be included in a balanced meal. A balanced meal, for instance, might contain vegetables, whole grains, and a serving of lean protein.

- Limit the size of portions: Controlling portion sizes is essential when meal planning. Using spoons and measuring cups to portion foods is one approach. The person's hand size can also be used to estimate portion sizes. A serving of protein, for instance, ought to be about the size of their palm.

- Serve a wide range of foods: Seniors get a variety of nutrients from foods that are offered. Additionally, it may enhance mealtime enjoyment. There should be a wide range of flavors and textures in a well-balanced meal.

- Take into account your calorie requirements: Seniors need different amounts of calories based on their age, gender, and level of activity. When planning meals, it's important to take these things into account. A registered dietitian can help you figure out how many calories you need.

You can ensure that seniors get the nutrients they need without overeating by planning meals that are balanced and taking portion sizes into consideration. Offering a variety of foods can also increase mealtime enjoyment.

Desserts and Snacks

Desserts and snacks can be a great way to give older people more food. For the elderly, here are some quick and healthy recipes for snacks and desserts:

- Parfait de yogurt: For a delicious and nutritious snack, layer granola and fresh fruit on top of low-fat yogurt.

- Trail Mix: For a nutrient-dense, portable snack, combine dark chocolate, nuts, seeds, dried fruits, and other ingredients.

- Crackers and cheese: Whole-grain crackers and low-fat cheese make a filling and satisfying snack.

- Apple Baked: Cut an apple and sprinkle with cinnamon and a modest quantity of earthy colored sugar. Make a dessert that is cozy and warm by baking it in the oven.

- Pops of frozen fruit: For a healthy dessert, puree fresh fruit with a little honey and freeze it in popsicle molds.

- Avocado and chocolate pudding: Combine avocado, cocoa powder, and honey to make a rich, creamy, and nutrient-dense dessert.

While picking tidbits and pastries for the older, taking into account their dietary limitations and individual needs is significant. Seniors with difficulty chewing, for instance, may require soft or pureed options, and diabetics may need to reduce their sugar intake.

By giving simple and nutritious tidbit and treat choices, you can assist with supporting the general wellbeing and prosperity of the old.

why snacks and desserts can be important for the elderly.

There are a number of reasons why snacks and desserts can be important for the elderly. Right off the bat, as we age, our cravings and appetite signs can change, making it more hard to consume an adequate number of supplements over the course of the day. Snacks can help make up for missing meals by providing extra calories and nutrients.

Additionally, dental issues, digestive issues, or other health conditions may make it difficult for many elderly people to consume larger meals.

Snacks can make it simple and convenient for them to get the nutrients they need without putting too much strain on their digestive systems.

Even though desserts aren't necessary for a healthy diet, they can be included in the elderly's diet. Desserts can be a source of pleasure, which is especially important for seniors who may be struggling with depression or isolation.

It is essential to keep in mind that desserts and snacks should be selected with care to ensure that they provide sufficient nutrition without being overly loaded with calories, sugar, or unhealthy fats. Snacks and desserts can be beneficial components of a healthy diet for the elderly if they are limited in portion sizes and made up of nutrient-dense options like fresh fruits, nuts, and low-fat dairy products.

Recipes for easy, healthy snacks and desserts, including options for those with dietary restrictions or difficulty chewing

Here are some recipes for easy, healthy snacks and desserts, including options for those with dietary restrictions or difficulty chewing:

- Salad of Soft Fruits: For a tasty and simple snack, cut up soft fruits like bananas, pears, and peaches into small pieces and combine them with low-fat vanilla yogurt and some cinnamon.

- Pineapple and cottage cheese: Diced pineapple on top of low-fat cottage cheese makes a digestible snack that is high in protein and low in sugar.

- Smoothie with Chocolate Bananas: For a creamy, nutritious snack that will satisfy your sweet tooth, combine ripe bananas, low-fat milk, cocoa powder, and ice.

- Sweet Potato Mash: For a vitamin A-rich, flavorful snack, mash boiled sweet potatoes with a little butter and cinnamon. Greek Yogurt with Berries: For a high-protein, antioxidant-rich snack, drizzle honey over Greek yogurt and top with fresh berries.

- Sauce of Apples: By combining apples, cinnamon, and a small amount of water in a pot, you can make your own unsweetened apple sauce. For people who have trouble chewing, this snack is ideal because it is soft and delicious.

- Delicate Heated Pear: Pears can be sliced and baked, sprinkled with cinnamon, until soft and tender. This dessert is full of vitamins and fiber and is easy to chew.

Consider the dietary restrictions and individual requirements of the elderly when selecting snacks and desserts. For instance, seniors with diabetes might have to restrict their sugar consumption, while those with biting challenges might require gentler or pureed choices. You can support the overall health and well-being of the elderly by providing snacks and desserts that are simple to prepare and contain nutritious ingredients.

Tips for making the preparation and consumption of snacks and desserts easier for the elderly

The following are some suggestions for making the preparation and consumption of snacks and desserts easier for the elderly:

Pre-portion desserts and snacks: Snacks and desserts can be divided into smaller bags or containers to make it easier for seniors to grab a quick snack without having to measure or cut.

Choose options that are soft and easy to chew: Soft options like yogurt or mashed fruits can make snack and dessert time more enjoyable and less stressful for seniors with dental issues or difficulty chewing.

Make it easier to use the tools and utensils: Seniors may find it easier to consume snacks and desserts without difficulty if, for instance, they are provided with a small fork or spoon for cut-up fruit or a spoon or straw for smoothies.

Pre-plan and freeze: Getting ready tidbits and sweets quite a bit early and freezing them can make it more straightforward to have various choices close by without setting them up each day.

Concentrate on foods high in nutrients: Seniors can get the most out of their snacks and desserts without having to eat a lot by choosing ones that are high in vitamins, fiber, protein, and other nutrients.

You can help make dessert and snack time for the elderly more enjoyable and beneficial by considering these suggestions.

Healthy Eating and Meal Planning for Older People

In this chapter, we'll talk about healthy eating and meal planning for older people.

- Choose foods high in nutrients: Although our bodies require fewer calories as we get older, they still require essential nutrients. Seniors can maintain their health and well-being by choosing foods high in vitamins, minerals, and fiber.

- Aim for variety: Seniors can get a wide range of nutrients and avoid becoming bored with their diets by eating a variety of foods. Encourage seniors to try new foods like whole grains, lean proteins, healthy fats, and fruits and vegetables.

- Avoid processed foods and foods high in sugar: Additives and processed foods can be high in calories but low in nutrients, which can cause obesity and other health problems. Seniors should be encouraged to choose whole foods and to avoid snacks and drinks with sugar.

- Control your portions: Overeating can cause health problems and weight gain. Use smaller plates and bowls, measure serving sizes, and avoid second helpings to help seniors practice portion control.

- Keep hydrated: Seniors can suffer from dehydration, so it's important to encourage them to drink a lot of fluids every day. Herbal teas, low-fat milk, and water are all viable options.

- Preparation for meals: Seniors can save time and energy by planning and preparing meals in advance and making healthier choices. They should be encouraged to prepare the ingredients ahead of time, make a shopping list, and plan meals for the week.

- Take into account diet restrictions: Seniors may need to limit certain foods due to dietary restrictions or health conditions. Create a meal plan with them that still provides a balanced diet while still meeting their needs and preferences.

Seniors can support their overall health and well-being by eating a well-balanced and healthy diet by following these recommendation

Elderly meal planning and healthy eating habits

Healthy meal planning and eating habits are important for the elderly to keep their health and well-being. Some suggestions:

- Try different foods: Seniors who consume a variety of foods receive all of the necessary nutrients for proper body function. Whole grains, lean proteins, vegetables, and healthy fats are all included in this.

- Limit the size of portions: Encourage seniors to eat in moderation because overeating can result in weight gain and other health problems. Utilizing more modest plates and bowls and allotting serving sizes can help.

- Make meals ahead of time: Seniors can save time and energy by planning their meals ahead of time and making healthier choices. They should be encouraged to prepare the ingredients ahead of time, make a shopping list, and plan meals for the week.

- Take into account diet restrictions: Seniors may need to limit certain foods due to dietary restrictions or health conditions. Create a meal plan with them that still provides a balanced diet while still meeting their needs and preferences.

- Keep hydrated: Seniors can suffer from dehydration, so it's important to encourage them to drink a lot of fluids every day. Herbal teas, low-fat milk, and water are all viable options.

- Avoid processed foods and foods high in sugar: Additives and processed foods can be high in calories but low in nutrients, which can cause obesity and other health problems. Seniors should be encouraged to choose whole foods and to avoid snacks and drinks with sugar.

- Take care when eating: Encourage seniors to eat mindfully and in the moment. This means focusing on the food they are eating and avoiding distractions like television or phones. They may be able to enjoy their meals more and avoid overeating thanks to this.

By following these smart dieting propensities and feast arranging procedures, seniors can keep up with their wellbeing and prosperity and forestall constant infections.

Tips for elderly grocery shopping and food storage

Grocery shopping and food storage can be difficult, but the following strategies can assist:

- Make a grocery list: Encourage seniors to make a list of the foods they need before going to the grocery store. They may be able to stay focused and avoid making impulsive purchases thanks to this.

- Shop outside of peak times: Seniors can save time by shopping during off-peak hours and avoiding crowds and long lines. It might also make it simpler for them to get around the store and locate the things they require.

- Take into account curbside pickup or delivery: For seniors who have difficulty getting to the store or carrying heavy groceries, many grocery stores now offer delivery or curbside pickup services.

- Look for discounts for seniors: Make sure to inquire about whether senior discounts are available at any given grocery store.

- Select items that have a longer shelf life: While choosing food sources, pick things with a more extended time span of usability, like canned or frozen products of the soil, entire grains, and dried beans. These food sources can endure longer and be utilized in various feasts.

- Good food storage: In order to preserve the food's quality and safety, proper storage is crucial. Encourage seniors to consume perishable foods like meat and dairy products before they expire by storing them in the refrigerator or freezer.

- Date and label the food: Food can be labeled and dated to help seniors remember what they have and when it will expire. This can ensure that they are consuming safe, fresh foods and reduce food waste.

Seniors can make grocery shopping and food storage easier and more efficient by following these tips. They can also ensure that they have access to foods that are healthy and nutritious.

Ideas for getting family members and caregivers involved in meal planning and preparation

Getting family members and caregivers involved in meal planning and preparation can be a great way to make sure seniors eat well and get the help they need. Here are a few concepts:

- Planning meals together: Set aside some time to plan the week's meals with loved ones or caregivers. This may assist in ensuring that the meals are nutritious and well-balanced for the senior.

- Cooking together: Cooking with others can be a fun and social activity as well as an easier way to prepare meals. Chopping vegetables or stirring pots on the stove can be done with the assistance of family members or caregivers.

- Services that deliver meals: Think about using a meal delivery service that provides senior citizens with nutritious and healthy meals. Family members and caregivers may feel less pressure to plan and prepare meals on their own as a result.

- Dinners with a crowd: Family members and caregivers can benefit greatly from participating in meal planning and preparation through potluck dinners. The senior can enjoy a variety of foods because everyone can bring a dish to share.

- Demonstrations of cooking: Consider sorting out a cooking show or class for relatives and parental figures to learn new recipes and cooking strategies. For everyone involved, this can be a fun and educational experience.

- Sharing recipes: Encourage caregivers and family members to share their favorite recipes. New concepts and motivation for meal planning and preparation may result from this.

Seniors can get the social and nutritional support they need to keep a healthy and balanced diet by having family members and caregivers help plan and prepare meals.